MUSHROOM CULTIVATION FOR BEGINNERS

Cultivate Deliciousness in your home.

Roy Freeman

Table of Contents

Introduction

Salutations from the fascinating world of mushroom cultivation! In this book, "Mushroom Cultivation for Beginners," we will delve into the fascinating world of fungi and learn why cultivating mushrooms is not just a fun hobby but also a helpful and sustainable one.

Mushroom farming offers a distinctive and alluring opportunity for individuals seeking a relationship with nature and a reliable source of delicious meals. Growing mushrooms requires far less space than normal gardening, making it possible for those with small properties or even those who live in cities. Beyond this, those who are intrigued by the mysteries of mycology, the study of fungus, have a lot to look forward to.

Beyond what you put on the plate, there are several benefits to growing your mushrooms. By cultivating your fungus, you may choose the kind and quality of mushrooms you consume. You may produce rare and exotic species that aren't often seen in stores, and you'll know precisely what went into their development – no pesticides, no preservatives, just pure, fresh mushrooms full of flavor and nutrition.

Mushroom cultivation is another eco-friendly pastime. Fungi are nature's recyclers, breaking down organic waste to create nutrient-rich soil. By cultivating mushrooms, you can reduce food waste and build a more sustainable food system.

Like any other industry, mushroom cultivation is not without its misconceptions. We'll debunk some of these common myths and get you moving in the right direction. Whether your issue is that mushroom culture is too hard for novices or that you need a large, dark basement to get started, we'll address these concerns and provide you with clear, practical information to help you get your mushroom cultivation adventure off to a great start.

The next chapters will go through the foundations of mushroom cultivation, from selecting the right mushroom species to understanding the necessary tools and techniques. We'll guide you step-by-step through the process, demystifying the art of mushroom farming and allowing you to enjoy a bountiful harvest.

So whether you're a curious novice or an experienced gardener looking to expand your knowledge, "Mushroom Cultivation for Beginners" is your passport to the fascinating world of mushrooms. Let's go on this exciting journey together to discover the joys and advantages of growing your own delicious, nutritious mushrooms.

Chapter

I

Initial Point

No matter one's level of gardening experience, cultivating mushrooms is a fun and rewarding pastime that anybody can take part in. Whether you're a seasoned gardener looking to broaden your knowledge or a complete novice eager to learn about fungi, this book is your in-depth guide to getting started in the fascinating world of mushroom gardening.

The Influence of Mushrooms

Before delving into the intricacies of producing mushrooms, it's critical to recognize the significance and wonder of these extraordinary organisms. The world's ecosystems depend on mushrooms, which are frequently referred to as nature's recyclers. They help to maintain ecological balance by decomposing organic waste and replenishing the soil's essential nutrients.

Mushrooms have long been recognized for their culinary and medicinal properties in addition to their importance to ecology. They come in an amazing range of shapes, sizes, and flavors, making them a treasured component in many different cuisines. Many mushrooms are also recognized for their purported health benefits, which include boosting the immune system, reducing inflammation, and aiding with stress management.

Why Do You Grow Your Mushrooms?

While picking wild mushrooms is one option, there are several advantages to producing your own:

- **Safety and Control Come First**

  You can control the development environment and ensure that the mushrooms you harvest are safe to eat by producing your mushrooms. There won't be a chance that you'll accidentally collect dangerous or inedible species.

- **Taste and Frische**

  Homegrown mushrooms are unparalleled in terms of flavor and freshness. The moment you choose them, you may experience their full taste and fragrance, enhancing your culinary creations.

- **Selection**

In the horticultural sector, there are a wide variety of mushrooms to explore, each with unique characteristics. You may sample a wide range of flavors, from the earthy shiitake flavor to the nutty aroma of oyster mushrooms.

- **Sustainability**

You promote a more sustainable way of life by growing your mushrooms. Utilizing homegrown mushrooms rather than store-bought ones reduces the environmental effect of packaging and shipping.

- **Interaction and Education**

Growing mushrooms is a learning experience as well as a way to produce food. Mycology, or the study of fungus, will become clearer to you, and you'll develop a strong connection with nature.

What you'll need

It's essential to gather the necessary tools and materials before beginning your mission to cultivate mushrooms. Here is a little selection to get you started:

- **Expanding Media**

  The growing medium you choose depends on the kind of mushroom you wish to cultivate. Common substitutes include straw, compost, wood chips, and sawdust.

- **Spawn**

  Your mushroom "seed" is called spawn. The specified species of mushrooms have invaded the substrate. Your offspring may be made or purchased.

- **Packaging**

  To keep your spawn and growing media organized, you'll need bags or containers. These might be anything from plastic bags to containers specifically made for mushroom cultivation.

- **Airflow and Humidity**

  Exact humidity and ventilation levels are required for mushrooms to grow correctly. Depending on your growth method, you could need a humidifier, a fan, or a misting system.

- **Control of Temperature and Light**

  Mushrooms don't need direct sunlight to develop, but they still need the right temperature and illumination. Consider using a grow light system or finding a suitable location.

- **Sanitation Equipment**

To prevent infection, you'll need equipment for sterilizing your growing material and containers. You may do this with a pressure cooker or a pasteurization device.

In the chapters that follow, we'll go into the mechanics of cultivating a variety of mushroom species, step-by-step instructions, troubleshooting tips, and even more complicated ways. After reading this book, you'll be equipped with the knowledge and confidence you need to begin your mushroom-growing experience. So let's put on our work boots and grab our supplies to begin this exciting mycological expedition.

The Best Species of Mushrooms to Choose

Choosing the right kind of mushroom is an important first step in the fascinating world of mushroom gardening. Your success and enjoyment with mushroom growing as a novice will be significantly impacted by this decision. Since each mushroom species has unique requirements, growth characteristics, and preferences, it is essential to make an informed choice. This chapter discusses the factors you should consider when deciding on the best species of mushroom to cultivate.

Own preferences: You need to start with your preferences when selecting a species of mushroom. Do you have a go-to variety of edible mushrooms? You could wish to cultivate mushrooms with certain culinary or medicinal qualities. You may make choices and maintain motivation throughout the development process by being aware of your preferences.

Think about your level of experience as a farmer. If you are a complete newbie, it is advised to start with species that are tolerant and relatively straightforward to cultivate, such as oyster mushrooms or shiitake. As you gain experience, you may examine more complex species like reishi or maitake.

Resources Available to You: Take into account the resources you have. Different kinds of mushrooms could need varying amounts of space, tools, and humidity control. Determine how much time, money, and space you have to dedicate to mushroom cultivation. While some species thrive in more constrained, compact environments, others thrive in larger, more regulated ones.

Environment & Climate: Different sorts of conditions, especially in terms of humidity and temperature, are required for various species of mushrooms. Take a look at the ideal climatic parameters for the species that interest you and compare them to your local climate. While certain varieties of mushrooms may be cultivated inside controlled environments, others thrive in specific locations when left to their own devices.

Decide why you are cultivating mushrooms. Do you grow mushrooms for their use in food, medicine, or simply for fun? Since many species have unique tastes and medicinal properties, choose a species that will assist you in achieving those goals.

Availability of Spores or Spawn: Verify that finding spores or spawn, the chosen mushroom's equivalent of seeds, will not be difficult for you. Examine the availability of any mushrooms that could need specialized suppliers before making a decision.

When choosing a time range, take your time commitment to mushroom cultivation into account. Since various species mature at various rates, choose a species that matches your time frame and level of patience. Some mushrooms can be harvested in a few weeks, while others may take many months.

Over time, don't be afraid to investigate and try out other mushroom species. You may discover new favorites as you gain experience or master the techniques required to properly produce a variety of mushrooms.

Choosing the perfect mushroom species is an exciting and personal decision that might lead to a fun farming journey. By taking into account your preferences, skill level, available resources, purpose, climate, and other factors, you can make an informed selection that satisfies your needs and goals. Remember that cultivating mushrooms is both an art and a science and that if you have the right species available to you, your attempt will be both fruitful and satisfying.

A Growth-Friendly Environment Can Be Created

Setting up the best circumstances for development is the first step in successful mushroom cultivation. As a newbie, it is crucial to comprehend and meet these requirements since mushrooms are special animals that need certain conditions to flourish. This chapter will go over the key elements that influence the growth of mushrooms as well as how to create a conducive environment for your fungal friends.

Temperature

One of the key factors in the growth of mushrooms is temperature. Keep the temperature consistent and within the range that is ideal for the particular species of mushrooms you have chosen. Different types of mushrooms need various temperatures. Here are some tips:

You may explore the ideal temperature range for your specific mushroom species.

Use a thermometer to monitor the temperature in your growing area.

Consider using a heating or cooling system to maintain the appropriate temperature.

Humidity

Mushrooms need high humidity levels, often 90% or more, to thrive. A certain humidity level is necessary for the growth of mature fruiting bodies, primordia formation, and mycelial development. The ideal humidity level may be maintained as follows:

1. To monitor moisture levels, get a humidity meter.

2. Use a humidifier, a misting system, or a humidity tent to maintain the required humidity.

3. Steer clear of over-saturating the substrate to prevent the growth of mold.

Light

Although mushrooms, unlike plants, do not need light for photosynthesis, they do require some indirect light to begin pinning and fruiting. The best way to deliver the right amount of light is as follows:

1. Keep the light in your development area indirect or partial. Avoid direct sunlight since it might harm the mycelium.

2. A 12-hour light cycle is often sufficient for the vast majority of mushroom species.

3. Some species, like shiitake, benefit from a brief exposure to natural light to encourage fruiting.

Air Exchange Adequate

Air Exchange Adequate air exchange is necessary for maintaining optimum mushroom growth. It guarantees the removal of carbon dioxide (CO_2) and the replacement of oxygen in the mycelium and fruiting bodies. Use an exhaust fan or a passive ventilation system to circulate air in your growth area for optimal air exchange. Limit the amount of airflow you provide to prevent drying out the substrate.

Maintain a regular schedule of air exchanges, often many times each day.

The Foundation and Container

The suitable substrate and container may be used to provide an ideal growing environment:

1. Choose a substrate, such as hardwood sawdust, straw, or a ready-made combination, that is appropriate for the kind of mushroom you have chosen.

2. Make sure your containers are sterile and clean to prevent illness.

3. Use containers with enough drainage and ventilation to stop additional moisture from building up.

4. Creating a conducive atmosphere for your mushrooms to thrive is an essential part of efficient growing. By carefully regulating the temperature, humidity, light, air exchange, substrate, and containers, you can create the ideal environment for your fungal crop to flourish.

Chapter

2

A Mushroom's Life Cycle

Understanding the mushroom life cycle is essential for successful cultivation. The life cycle of mushrooms is intriguing and peculiar, consisting of several growth stages, each with specific requirements and characteristics. This chapter will go through the complicated life cycle of the mushroom, from spore to fruiting body, as well as the critical factors that influence development at each stage.

Spore Stage: A mushroom's life cycle begins with the spore stage. Spores, which are tiny, dust-like particles, are the mushrooms' reproductive organs. They are freed from mature mushroom caps and disperse over the area. Spores are very adaptable and can withstand extreme heat and dry conditions.

Germination

Upon landing on a suitable substrate, spores begin to proliferate when the conditions are favorable. During the germination process, a spore develops into a mycelium, a structure that resembles a thread. The mycelium, which makes up the vegetative component of the mushroom, is in charge of growth and nutrient absorption.

Mycelial Growth

As it spreads over the substrate, the mycelium consumes nutrients and breaks down organic matter. This stage may last for many weeks or even months, depending on the kind of mushroom and the climate. The ideal balance of temperature, humidity, and nutrient accessibility is crucial for the best mycelial growth.

Fundamental Formation

When the environment is perfect and the mycelium has fully colonized the substrate, it then moves on to the next stage, primordia development. During this stage, the formation of primordia, or "baby mushrooms," small pin-like structures, begins. These primordia are the developing fruiting bodies' embryonic forms.

Body Fruiting Growth

As they grow, the primordia evolve into fully formed fruiting bodies. What we often think of as mushrooms are the fruiting bodies, which resemble mushrooms. Mycelium focuses on spore production when the mushroom's cap and stem start to expand. The kind of mushroom and the surroundings affect the size and rate of growth of the mushrooms.

Spore Release

Fruiting bodies release spores into the environment after they are completely developed. The mushroom's life cycle is now finished, and the spores are ready for dissemination with the potential to resume the cycle if they land on a suitable substrate.

Understanding the fungus' life cycle is vital for growing mushrooms properly. By providing the appropriate conditions at each stage, mushroom growers may encourage healthy growth and boost their yields. Mushroom growing is an interesting and fulfilling pastime for both beginning and experienced growers since each step of the mushroom life cycle, from spore to fruiting body, presents its opportunities and challenges. In the following chapters, we'll go through the specific requirements and practices for producing a variety of mushroom species, giving you the knowledge you need to successfully begin your mushroom farming endeavor.

The Mold Life Cycle

The life cycle of mushrooms must first be understood by everyone who wishes to embark on the beautiful journey of mushroom development. Mushrooms have a well-defined life cycle, even though they may seem to be enigmatic organisms. In this chapter, we'll delve into the complexity of the fungi's life cycle and demystify all of its many stages, from spore to fully formed fruiting body.

Initial Stages of Spore Formation

A small component called a spore serves as the first step in the life cycle of a mushroom. These spores, which mimic seeds in plants, are the reproductive parts of fungus. Expelled from adult mushroom caps, they disperse across the vicinity and wait for the ideal conditions to germinate. Each spore contains genetic material unique to that particular species of mushroom.

Germination's Initial Stage

When the conditions are right, usually when there is adequate moisture and an appropriate substrate, spores begin to germinate. During the germination process, a single spore develops into a hypha, a structure like a thread. With this hypha, a new mycelium is beginning.

Mycelium Development: The Vegetative Stage

A small component called a spore serves as the first step in the life cycle of a mushroom. The mushroom's vegetative portion is called the mycelium.

It is made up of a vast network of hyphae that ingest nutrients from the substrate and penetrate it. The formation of the fungal mycelium, which prepares the organism for reproduction, is an important phase in the fungal life cycle. As it develops, the mycelium secretes enzymes to degrade organic materials and provide nutrition for the fungus.

The Knot's Hidden Meaning: The Promise of Mushrooms

Once the mycelium has consumed enough nutrients and the conditions are right, it enters a phase known as knot production. At this stage, the mycelium begins to divide, forming tiny knots known as primordia. On the substrate, these knots, which signify the first stages of mushroom development, are often seen as small pinlike forms.

Developing Fruiting Bodies: The Mushroom Appearance

Rapidly expanding primordia ultimately develop into fruiting bodies that we harvest as mushrooms. The pili (cap) and the stipe (stalk) make up the fruiting bodies. As the mushrooms develop, the cap expands and they reach their full size. At this point, the distinctive qualities of the mushroom species you are cultivating will become clear.

Spore Spread: The Cycle Continues

After the adult mushroom excreta, the life cycle comes full circle. After being scattered by the wind or another force, the spores may land on other surfaces and re-ignite the germination process. This continual cycle ensures the survival of the fungus species.

Selecting Substrates

Choosing the right substrate is one of the most crucial aspects of the mushroom-growing process. Substrates are what feed mushrooms, giving them the essential nutrients they need to grow and thrive. Being able to choose the right substrates will be essential to your success as a beginner in mushroom growing. In this chapter, we'll look at the many factors you should consider while selecting substrates, helping you make decisions, and assuring a successful and plentiful harvest.

Understanding the Materials

Before diving into the specifics of substrate selection, it is essential to understand what substrates are and why they are important in the mushroom-growing process. Substrates are essentially the items or situations in which mushrooms may grow. These elements provide mushrooms nourishment and create an atmosphere that is conducive to their growth. The substrate you choose will have a significant influence on the kind and quantity of mushrooms you may produce.

Considerations to Make When Selecting Substrates

Various species of mushrooms each have a favored substrate. Oyster mushrooms (Pleurotus spp.) may grow on a variety of lignocellulosic materials, including straw and coffee grounds, whereas shiitake mushrooms (Lentinula edodes) are similar to hardwood sawdust. Before choosing a substrate, choose one that is appropriate for the kinds of mushrooms you wish to cultivate.

Cost and Availability: Consider the price and supply of substrates in your region. While certain substrates can be simple to get and affordable, others might be difficult to locate or expensive. Consider your budget and the resources in your region while choosing your substrate.

The necessary nutrients should be present in the substrate to promote the growth of mushrooms. Nutrient-rich soils often provide higher harvests. Nutritional supplies including minerals, nitrogen, and carbohydrates are common. For instance, soybean hulls and wheat straws are excellent sources of nitrogen and carbohydrates.

A sanitary environment must be maintained for mushrooms to develop well. The susceptibility of various substrates to contamination varies. Before beginning, take into account the substrate's sterility and take precautions to minimize the risk of infection.

Water Retention Capacity: The ability of a substrate to retain moisture is essential for the growth of mushrooms. Mushrooms need a steady supply of moisture to grow. Strong water-holding substrates may help to maintain appropriate moisture levels throughout the cultivation phase.

pH Level: Different species of mushrooms need different pH levels. While some mushrooms like somewhat acidic substrates, others thrive better in more alkaline settings. The pH of your substrate should be adjusted as required to fit the kind of mushrooms you've chosen.

Pre-processing Requirements: Some substrates must be pre-processed, such as by pasteurization or sterilization, to get rid of competitors and provide an optimum environment for mushroom mycelium. Prepare yourself for these additional steps while selecting substrates.

How do Substances function?

In the context of mushroom cultivation, the material on which mushrooms grow is referred to as a substrate. It serves as the medium that provides the mycelium, the vegetative part of the fungus, with the sustenance and assistance it needs to colonize and eventually develop fruiting bodies (the mushrooms). Imagine it as mushroom soil, except we use a range of organic or synthetic components to create a fungus-friendly environment.

The idea of "substrate" is essential to the success of your efforts in the field of mushroom cultivation. Regardless of your level of experience or if you are just starting, understanding substrates and how they work is crucial. In this chapter, we'll look at the concept of substrates and how crucial they are to the growth of mushrooms.

Various Substances

For mushroom culture, a variety of substrates may be utilized, and the choice of substrate often depends on the kind of mushroom you wish to grow. Here are a few examples of common substrates:

Shiitake and oyster mushrooms are two types of mushrooms that like to grow on woody surfaces like oak or beech. Wood-based substrates are typically prepared by cutting or grinding the wood into small pieces and then nutrient-adding it.

Many different kinds of mushrooms, particularly the White Button mushroom, grow well on straw-based substrates. It is readily available and may be blended with other foods to boost their nutritional value.

A few grains that may be used as substrates include rye, millet, or wheat. To give the mycelium time to colonize before being transferred to a bulk substrate, they are often employed for the production of spawn.

Manure-Based Substrates: Psilocybe cubensis and other mushroom species thrive on manure-based substrates because they provide essential nutrients. Horse and cow dung are often used.

Used coffee grounds are an alternative for home gardeners looking for a substrate. They may be used as supplements to other materials to increase their nutritional value.

Sawdust: When nutrient-supplemented, sawdust is excellent for producing several wood-loving mushroom species.

Advanced culture allows for the cultivation of certain mushroom species on synthetic substrates made from various chemical components.

Choosing the right substrate is crucial since various mushroom species have different preferences for their growth conditions. You must match the substrate to the kind of mushrooms you want to cultivate for it to be successful.

Create the Foundation

Substrate preparation is a critical step in the mushroom-growing process. To eliminate competing germs that can obstruct the growth of mushrooms, sterilization or pasteurization is required. When preparing the substrate, the correct pH level, moisture content, and nutritional balance must all be considered.

Common Bases for Different Mushroom Species

One of the key components of success in the fascinating world of mushroom cultivation is choosing the right substrate for your chosen type of mushroom. The substrate is the material that mushrooms grow on and get their essential nutrients from. Effective mushroom growth requires an understanding of the unique substrate requirements of different mushroom species. We'll discuss common substrates for various mushroom types as you start your mushroom production journey to provide you with the knowledge you need to make informed choices.

Toggle Mushrooms

Button mushrooms, often known as white mushrooms or champignons, are among the most widely cultivated mushrooms worldwide. Compost that is rich in organic matter is ideal for them. Typical substrates for button mushrooms include the following:

1. Horse manure, straw, gypsum, and other organic materials are the primary substrate for button mushrooms.

2. It is a sustainable choice since any compost that is left over after a crop of button mushrooms has been harvested may be utilized to make additional compost.

3. Shiitake mushrooms are regarded for their umami flavor and medicinal properties. These mushrooms are often seen growing on hardwood logs or sawdust-based substrates.

Typical substrates for shiitake mushrooms include:

1. Hardwood logs: Oak, beech, and maple are your best bets. It is necessary to add shiitake mycelium to the logs.

2. Hardwood sawdust and wood chips mixed with shiitake spawn are often used for indoor cultivation.

Oyster Mushrooms of the Pleurotus Species

Oyster mushrooms are known for their colorful variety of delicate, fan-shaped caps. They are flexible and may develop on a variety of substrates, including:

Straw that has been pasteurized is a preferred substrate for oyster mushrooms. It often has gypsum or bran added to it to provide more nutrients.

Coffee grounds: It's a sustainable decision to use used coffee grounds as a substrate for the development of oyster mushrooms.

Cardboard: Cardboard may be shredded and used as a substrate for small-scale indoor gardening.

Enoki mushrooms are also referred to as Flammulina velutipes.

Due to their long, thin stems and small caps, enoki mushrooms need cool temperatures. They often grow up eating a variety of:

Wheat straw: Pasture-grown wheat straw is often used as a substrate for enoki mushrooms.

Sawdust: Wheat straw's texture and nutritional value could be enhanced by adding hardwood sawdust to it.

Mushroom with Lions' Manes

For its potential health benefits, lion's mane-shaped mushrooms are highly desired. They often develop on surfaces with a hardwood basis:

1. Hardwood sawdust: The mycelium that gives lions their manes is often produced using bran and hardwood sawdust.

2. Logs: Like shiitake mushrooms, lion's mane may be cultivated on hardwood logs.

Remember that for the best possible mushroom production, adequate substrate preparation, cleanliness, and environmental conditions are necessary. Even though these are common substrates for many types of mushrooms, as your mushroom output improves, exploration and variety may lead to exciting discoveries. Every variety of mushrooms has various requirements, so do your research and follow the regulations for the best outcomes. Happy mushroom growing!

Maintaining Sanitary Conditions

Maintaining sanitary conditions is essential for mushroom production. How well you produce mushrooms will depend on your ability to prevent pollution. Contaminants might kill your mushroom cultures, putting your whole harvest in peril. In this chapter, we'll go over the essential techniques and processes that will help you maintain sterile conditions throughout growing mushrooms.

The Value of Fertility: There are no potentially harmful contaminants or microorganisms in a sterile environment. Because it ensures that only the desired mushroom mycelium grows and prevents the invasion of competing organisms, sterility is crucial for mushroom cultivation. Maintaining sterility improves harvest prospects and lowers the risk of infection.

Before entering your cultivation area, it's necessary to practice good personal cleanliness. Think about putting on fresh, long-sleeved clothing and doing a complete handwashing with soap and water. A hairnet and a pair of disposable gloves are practical additions to your attire.

Your workspace should be neat and free of clutter, dust, and other obstructions. Maintain the cleanliness and sterility of all surfaces, utensils, and equipment you'll be using for mushroom cultivation.

Laminar Flow Hood or Glove Box: A laminar flow hood or glove box is a smart investment to maintain hygienic conditions. These gadgets provide a controlled environment where the air is filtered and sterilized before it reaches your desk, reducing the risk of infection. For novices, a laminar flow hood could be more practical.

Clean up Your Substance and Your Containers: Clean your substrate completely before introducing mycelium or mushroom spores. Sterilization methods including steam baths, autoclaving, and pressure cooking are often used. Containers like jars and sacks should also be sanitized to prevent infection.

Inoculation Technique: When injecting spores or mycelium into the substrate, it's critical to apply the proper inoculation techniques. Use a flame-sterilized inoculation tool (such as a needle or scalpel) to transfer the culture. Work quickly but carefully to minimize the length of time the substrate is exposed to potential contaminants.

Ventilation and air filtration: If a laminar flow hood is not available, you may utilize a high-efficiency particulate air (HEPA) filter in your growing environment. As a result, air pollution will be reduced. Aim for adequate circulation and ventilation while preventing drafts that might introduce contaminants.

Get Rid of Contaminated Cultures: Despite your best efforts, contamination may still occur. As soon as contamination is found in one culture, it should be isolated to prevent it from spreading to other cultures. Be sure to dispose of dangerous items properly.

Regular Cleaning and Maintenance: Maintaining a clean environment is an ongoing task. Regularly sterilize and clean your workspace, tools, and equipment. Change or clean your air filters as needed, keep an eye out for any potential sources of pollution, and take care of them.

The maintenance of hygienic conditions is essential for efficient mushroom production. By practicing great personal hygiene, utilizing the proper equipment, and strictly adhering to sterilizing and inoculation methods, you may dramatically reduce the risk of infection and increase your chances of getting a bountiful mushroom crop. It's crucial to remember that refining the art of sterile mushroom cultivation takes time and careful attention to detail.

Chapter

3

Incubation

It takes time to grow successfully in the fascinating world of mushroom gardening. Like all living things, mushrooms need certain conditions and a carefully controlled environment to flourish. A crucial step in the creation of mushrooms is incubation. This chapter covers the importance of incubation, the components required, and how to ensure that your mushroom project gets off to a strong start.

How Significant Is Incubation?

The incubation stage is an important one in the life cycle of mushrooms since it comes after the inoculation or spawning stage and before the fruiting stage. At this stage, the substrate is colonized by the mycelium, the fungus' vegetative part. This colonization process is significant for several reasons:

Substrate Colonization: Due to mycelium proliferation, the substrate might be colonized. For the absorption of nutrients and, finally, the development of robust, healthy fruiting bodies, this colonization is crucial.

Contaminants that Compete: The risk that the mycelium may get polluted by undesired fungus or bacteria is decreased by providing it with the ideal home. Contaminants could prevent mushrooms from growing and reduce your production.

Creating Ideal Situations: Stable temperatures and humidity levels are essential for the mycelium's growth and health, and you may control these factors during incubation. Frequently, these needs are different from those that apply during the fruiting phase.

Factors Affecting Incubation

To complete a healthy incubation period, it is important to carefully consider several factors:

Temperature: For a wide variety of mushroom species, a range of temperatures is optimal during incubation. Temperatures between 75°F and 80°F (24°C and 27°C) are good for many common mushroom varieties.

Humidity: Maintaining high humidity levels (about 90%) is necessary to prevent the substrate from drying out and to encourage mycelial growth.

Although mycelium thrives in conditions of high humidity, it also requires the movement of fresh air to prevent the production of poisonous gases and to encourage healthy development. Periodically, a controlled exchange of air is required.

Light: Unlike during the fruiting stage, the incubation stage of mushrooms does not need light. Mycelium may suffer from light exposure because it could encourage the growth of harmful microorganisms.

Increasing the Success of the Incubator

Follow these essential procedures to ensure a good incubation phase in your mushroom cultivation endeavor:

1. Keep the environment consistent: Keep an eye on and maintain the right temperatures and humidity levels during the incubation period. Investing in high-quality thermometers and hygrometers is essential.

2. Make sure there is enough fresh air exchange while preventing contamination or drafts. A simple air exchange system with filters may be employed to achieve this balance.

3. Keep calm: The length of the incubation period may range from a few days to many weeks, depending on the kind of mushroom and environmental conditions. Be patient and avoid hurrying the process.

4. Maintain strict cleanliness standards while handling your substrate and equipment to lower the risk of infection.

Incubation is a critical step in mushroom cultivation that establishes the circumstances for optimal fruiting and a large crop. By understanding the importance of incubation and properly managing the factors involved, you may effectively grow mushrooms. The following chapter discusses the exciting transition from the incubation to the fruiting phase as well as the techniques you must learn to develop your mushrooms to maturity.

Creating the Perfect Incubation Environment

Creating and maintaining the ideal circumstances for your fungal friends to thrive is frequently key to success in the world of mushroom farming. Creating the right incubation conditions is the critical next step after inoculating your substrate with mushroom spores or mycelium. This chapter will show you how to create the perfect incubation conditions to ensure a large mushroom harvest.

Understanding Incubation

Mycelium colonizes the substrate and builds a substantial web of threads during the incubation stage of mushroom production. This stage is crucial for the development of a strong and healthy mushroom culture. Because your mushrooms are vulnerable to contamination while they are incubating, it is essential to create a controlled environment that encourages mycelial growth while discouraging unwanted competitors.

Things that Influence Incubation

Several variables are taken into account while designing the appropriate incubation conditions, including:

- **Thermostat**

Mushrooms are temperature-sensitive organisms. The ideal temperature for incubation varies depending on the kind of mushroom, although it normally falls between 75°F and 80°F (24°C and 27°C). Maintaining a steady temperature within this range is vital to ensuring that the mycelium grows aggressively.

Moisture maintaining ideal humidity levels is equally important. An ideal incubation environment for the majority of mushroom species is a relative humidity of around 95%. This may be achieved by spraying the growing region or using a humidifier. Strong mycelial growth is promoted by constant moisture levels, which also keep the substrate from drying out.

- **Light**

During incubation, mycelium does not need light. By exposing your growing medium to light, you run the risk of encouraging the growth of harmful organisms. Keep the incubation chamber dark and save the light for the fruiting period.

- ## Switch, Air

Although mycelium does not need oxygen in the same manner as mushrooms do, it does need some air exchange to prevent the production of poisonous gases. In excess, carbon dioxide, which is generated during fungal respiration, may be toxic. To give a little air exchange, use filtered air exchange equipment or manually fan your growing containers.

- ## Neatness

It is crucial to maintain the incubation area's cleanliness. This helps prevent bacterial, fungal, or competing microbial infections. Use hygienic practices while handling your mushroom culture, such as washing your hands thoroughly and sterilizing your utensils.

- ## Building of the Incubation Chamber

To provide the optimal incubation circumstances, you may set up a customized incubation chamber or use a method that works for your growing area:

DIY Incubator: You may make an incubator out of basic materials like a large plastic storage container, a thermometer, and a small humidifier. This makes it possible for you to monitor and control the humidity and temperature of the container.

Built-In Incubators: You might also purchase pre-made incubation chambers made specifically for growing mushrooms. They often include built-in humidity and temperature controls for convenience.

- ## Observation and Adjustment

Regularly check the temperature, humidity, and cleanliness of the incubation chamber. To maintain the optimal conditions, adjust as required. While researching your incubation setup, take into account the unique requirements that different mushroom species may have, and make alterations as required.

For beginners, creating proper incubation conditions is a crucial step in the creation of mushrooms. By paying strict attention to temperature, humidity, cleanliness, and air exchange, you can provide your mushroom mycelium the ideal environment for development. The following chapter will go through the exciting process from incubation to fruiting when your mushrooms will finally become visible for harvest.

- ## Monitoring Mycelial Growth

For mushrooms to be effectively grown, mycelial growth must be watched carefully. Understanding the establishment and development of the mycelium, the fungus-based network that serves as the foundation for mushroom development is essential to guaranteeing a bountiful harvest. The importance of monitoring mycelial growth is covered in detail in this chapter, along with practical advice and techniques.

- ## The Value of Monitoring Mycelial Growth

Watching the Mycelial Growth By monitoring mycelial growth, you can keep an eye on how your endeavor to produce mushrooms is progressing. It allows you to assess if your mycelium is healthy and progressing as expected or whether there are issues that need attention.

Early detection of contamination: Contamination may substantially impede the development of mushrooms. You may spot contamination early on and take necessary steps to stop it from spreading by regularly observing the mycelial growth.

Environmental Conditions Optimization Mycelial growth is influenced by environmental factors like as temperature, humidity, and light. By monitoring growth, you may adjust these elements to create the ideal habitat for your mushrooms.

- ## Watching for Mycelial Growth

Visual Examination: Regularly inspect the mycelium in your substrate or spawn. Mycelium that is in good health should be white, fluffy, and spread widely. Any changes in color, texture, or the presence of strange growths might be signs of a problem.

Smell your mycelium to check for cleanliness and earthiness. Pollution may be indicated by unpleasant smells. Try using your sense of smell as a warning system.

Observe how quickly the mycelium colonizes the substrate. The kind of mushroom and the environment may have an impact on this rate. By monitoring this measure, you can forecast when your substrate will be ready for the next stage of growing.

Pay attention to the density and texture of the mycelium. It must be consistent and uniform across the substrate. Unusual behaviors might be a symptom of problems like drying out or having too much moisture.

Conduct a contamination check: Look out for any signs of contamination, such as discordant hues, atypical growths, or bad odors. As soon as you notice infection, confine the infected area.

Photography-based documentation Take photos of your mycelium at various phases of growth. This visual record might be used as a reference and to troubleshoot.

How to Address Mycelial Growth Issues

Slow Growth: If mycelial growth is too slow, you may wish to modify the environment or choose a more active strain of mycelium.

Aggressive Contamination: If it spreads fast, separate the contaminated area and discard it. Your workplace and equipment should be cleaned and sanitized to prevent the spread of illness.

If your mycelium exhibits odd hues or textures, check the specific mushroom species you're cultivating to see if there are any potential issues.

The ability to monitor mycelial development is among the most crucial for any aspiring mushroom farmer to possess. You may use it to check on the health of your mycelium, spot issues as they arise, and ultimately raise your chances of a successful mushroom harvest. By making frequent observations and changes to the environment, you may develop into a proficient mushroom farmer who can reliably produce high-quality mushrooms.

Troubleshooting Common Issues

Congratulations on beginning your mushroom farming journey! It's typical for a newcomer to have some setbacks along the way. In this part, we'll look at some common issues that mushroom growers deal with and provide solutions to help you get beyond them. If you run across problems, don't give up since every obstacle is an opportunity to improve. Let's begin addressing common issues in mushroom growing.

- **Development of Mold**

Mold growth on your substrate or mushrooms that is not wanted.

The ideal strategy is to maintain a clean and hygienic environment during the growth period. Ensure that your workspace, tools, and hands are all clean. Use sterility while inoculating substrate jars or bags. To encourage the development of mushrooms rather than mold, adjust ventilation and humidity levels.

- **Bacteria Contamination**

Issue: foul odor, slimy substrate, or discolored mycelium.

Solution: Follow sterilizing procedures exactly, use clean water, and make sure there is ample airflow. Limit crowding and dispose of contaminated substrates quickly.

- **Temperature Variations**

Problem: Slow or stagnant mycelium growth.

Solution: Monitor the temperature and keep it within the range recommended by the specific mushroom species you are using. As required, use heated pads, thermostats, or cooling measures.

- **Humidity Problems**

Problem: Insufficient or excessive humidity prevents fruiting.

Solution: To control humidity levels, use a humidifier, a humidifier, or enough ventilation. A hygrometer may be used to measure humidity appropriately.

- **Minor issues**

  Problem: Fruiting cannot be triggered due to improper lighting conditions.

  Solution: Ensure that your kind of mushrooms receives the proper illumination. While most need indirect or diffused illumination, there are certain times when complete darkness is required.

- **Availability of Dry Support**

  Problem: Mushroom growth is hampered by a dry substrate.

  Maintain the substrate's optimal moisture levels by sprinkling it or adding water as needed. Use a substrate mix that is appropriate for the kind of mushrooms you are growing.

- **Under-crushed Substrate**

  Poor fruiting and sluggish mycelium colonization are problems.

  Solution: Loosen your substrate mixture to enhance airflow and mycelium growth. Avoid packing it too firmly.

The environment in the fruiting chamber

Issue: Unpredictable conditions in the fruiting chamber.

Solution: To maintain a constant environment, utilize a humidifier, heater, or cooling system depending on your mushroom's requirements. Maintain consistent monitoring and adjusting of environmental parameters.

Although it may be educational and entertaining, growing mushrooms can sometimes be challenging. Remember that you must be persistent, pay close attention to detail, and always learn new things if you want to be successful as a mushroom farmer. By accurately identifying and correcting common issues, you'll develop your skills and increase your chances of harvesting a bountiful crop. As you work to learn the art, be composed and seek out advice from knowledgeable mushroom growers or other sources.

Chapter

4

Harvesting and Fruiting

Greetings, novice mushroom grower! You have finished all of the processes required to cultivate mushrooms, including choosing the ideal substrate and inoculating and incubating the species you want to grow. Now that fruiting and mushroom harvesting are here, the most exciting part of the journey has begun. In this chapter, you will be guided through the steps and factors that must be taken into account for a successful harvest.

The Fruit Production

Your attempts to cultivate mushrooms will bear fruit. At this point, mushrooms are produced by your mycelium network and they begin to expand and flourish. To ensure a good fruiting process, do the following steps:

Environmental Settings

By frequently misting or using a humidity chamber, you may keep the humidity level high (between 90 and 95%). The right amount of humidity is necessary for the development of mushrooms.

Depending on the kind of mushroom, maintain a moderate temperature. Typically, the ranges are between 13°C and 24°C, or 55°F and 75°F.

Clear, Bright Air

Mushrooms need light to begin pinning and establish a day-night cycle. However, they don't need direct sunlight. Use a soft, indirect light source, such as LED or fluorescent lighting, wherever possible. Additionally, you should provide fresh air by fanning or using an air exchange system to promote healthy mushroom growth.

Pinning

The substrate surface begins to grow tiny mushroom pins during the pinning stage. Your mushrooms are ready to begin growing once this occurs. Make sure your substrate surface is clean, damp, and impure-free to encourage consistent pinning.

The Development of Mushrooms

Once developed, pins will quickly grow into mature mushrooms. Keep a close eye on them and keep an eye on the humidity and temperature levels. Be patient since different mushroom species grow at different speeds.

How to Collect Mushrooms

The awaited moment has come: harvesting. Mushrooms need to be picked at the right moment to improve their quality and yield. How to accomplish it is as follows:

Tempo

Mushrooms are ready to be picked after the caps have fully opened but before the gills start to release spores. Ripe mushrooms may lose some of their flavor and texture if you wait too long. Harvest them by gently twisting or cutting them at the stem's base.

Tools

Use a clean, razor-sharp knife or a pair of scissors to cut the mushrooms. Avoid using your hands to prevent infection or injury. Organize your collected mushrooms in a spotless basket or container.

Neatness

Maintain sterility in the region during harvesting. Put on clean gloves and make sure your harvesting equipment is disinfected to prevent infection.

Regular Harvesting

Several mushroom species are capable of many flushes. After the first harvest, monitor your substrate and maintain the right conditions so that more mushrooms may grow. Some species may produce several flushes over many weeks.

When all your hard work pays off, the periods of mushroom growth known as fruiting and harvesting are the most gratifying. By creating the right environment and timing your harvests correctly, you may enjoy a copious crop of delicious, local mushrooms. In the next chapter, we'll go over the importance of proper storage and post-harvest care to preserve the life and quality of your treasured crop.

Happy Mushroom Growing!

Disclaimer: Always follow safety regulations and legislation while cultivating mushrooms. For information on the requirements of the particular kind of mushrooms you have chosen, you should also consult specialized resources.

Beginning of the Fruiting Stage

Dear reader, congrats on reaching this significant point in your mushroom gardening journey. By this time, your mycelium has grown effectively, you've seen it colonize a substrate, and you've seen how your inoculated substrate or substrate used in a mushroom grow kit develops into a strong fungal network. The pleasant and visually beautiful vegetative stage must give way to the fruiting period.

Understanding the Fruiting Stage

The much-awaited mushrooms begin to develop when the mushroom-growing process reaches the fruiting stage, which occurs after the mycelium has conquered the substrate. This step in the cultivation process is crucial, and it requires certain conditions and care to ensure a productive yield. Here is a rundown of what happens at this point:

When the right conditions are present, the mycelium starts to generate primordia, which are tiny mushroom pegs. These needles, which are often small, white, and scarcely noticeable, represent the first phases of mushroom development.

Mushroom Growth: As the primordia mature, they swiftly develop into adult mushrooms. It will start to resemble the familiar mushroom caps and stems.

When the mushrooms have reached the right size and maturity, they may be harvested. When harvesting, care should be taken to protect the mycelium and any potential for future fruiting.

Many Flushes: A type of mushroom may generate several flushes of mushrooms if the ideal conditions are available.

Environmental Factors That Affect Mushroom Fruiting

One of the key requirements for effective mushroom cultivation is the creation of appropriate environmental conditions for fruiting. The growth of mushrooms from their mycelium to fully formed fruiting bodies requires certain environmental conditions. Mushrooms are unique animals. This chapter will discuss the essential environmental factors for mushroom fruiting to assist novices in becoming knowledgeable mushroom farmers.

Temperature: The proper temperature must be maintained for mushrooms to fruit. The bulk of mushrooms require temperatures between 55°F and 75°F (13°C and 24°C), while various varieties of mushrooms have varying optimal temperatures. You must have a solid understanding of the specific temperature needs of the variety of mushrooms you are cultivating and keep your environment constant within those limits. Consistent temperature promotes proper fruiting and prevents heat stress on the mycelium.

Conditions with high humidity are optimal for growing mushrooms. During the fruiting phase, a humidity level of around 90% is suitable for the vast majority of mushroom species. The high relative humidity encourages the development of healthy, mature mushrooms by preventing the developing fruiting bodies from drying up. Using a humidifier or misting system as a source of humidity allows you to effectively control the humidity levels.

Mushrooms are fairly sensitive to light, even though they do not need it for photosynthesis in the same way that plants do. Several different mushroom species are stimulated to produce fruiting bodies by low ambient light levels. However, direct sunlight should be avoided since it may dry up the soil and stop the fruit from maturing. Direct, diffused natural light or low-intensity artificial light may be beneficial.

Air Exchange: A certain amount of air exchange is necessary for mushrooms to grow. Both the formation of fruiting bodies and mycelial respiration need oxygen. The mycelium creates carbon dioxide (CO2), which must be expelled to prevent it from accumulating. Use vents or an exhaust fan to aid in the elimination of CO2 and the intake of fresh air. Because of consistent air exchange, mushrooms develop healthily.

Conditions of the Substrate: The substrate, on which your mushroom mycelium grows, has a significant impact on fruiting. The moisture content, texture, and composition of the substrate should be suitable for the specific mushroom species you are cultivating. Correctly pasteurized or sterilized substrate materials also help to avoid contamination, which might obstruct fruiting.

Fruiting Chamber: A customized fruiting chamber has to be constructed to control the fruiting environment. This chamber should maintain the ideal levels of temperature, humidity, and air exchange for your chosen mushroom species. Typical options for fruiting chambers include growing tents, plastic containers, and specialty mushroom fruiting chambers.

Patience and timing: Finally, it's critical to have patience and understand the mushroom's life cycle. Given that various species have varied fruiting seasons, research is required to understand when to expect fruiting. Rushing the process might lead to poor crops or low yields.

To obtain optimal mushroom fruiting, environmental factors must be properly taken into account. By maintaining the ideal temperature, humidity, light, air exchange, and substrate conditions as well as using a customized fruiting chamber, beginners may provide the best conditions for mushroom growth. Always research the unique requirements that each mushroom species may have, then adapt your approach accordingly. If you have the right knowledge and patience, you can grow healthy and plentiful mushroom harvests.

Harvesting Procedures

Congratulations on your great mushroom growth! The moment has come to learn about the crucial component of mushroom gardening, and harvesting, now that your mushrooms have grown to their full potential. A vital part of mushroom growing is harvesting, and doing it properly will guarantee that you get the most enjoyment out of your hard work. We will examine numerous methods and recommendations for gathering mushrooms safely and successfully in this chapter.

Management of time

Before beginning your harvest, it is essential to determine when your mushrooms are ready to be harvested. The time varies according to the kind of mushroom, however, there are a few common indications to look out for:

Size: Mushrooms are typically ready to be picked when they reach the appropriate size. Shiitake mushrooms are harvested when their caps have fully developed, unlike button mushrooms, which are typically harvested when they are 1 to 2 inches in diameter.

Another useful indicator is the mushroom cap's color. Keep an eye out for any changes in color since mushrooms often change color as they develop.

Look at the gills or holes beneath the cap of the mushroom. They reach full maturity around the time of harvest.

Tools You'll Need

The following typical tools are required to collect mushrooms:

Make sure you use a clean, sharp knife or pair of scissors to correctly cut the mushroom stems.

Use a basket or container to collect the collected mushrooms without inflicting any harm.

Gloves: Although it is not necessary, using gloves may help keep your mushrooms clean and pathogen-free.

Harvesting Techniques

Harvesting techniques for various kinds of mushrooms should be slightly different:

Shiitake mushrooms: Gently twist the mushroom cap to separate it from the stem. Pulling too hard might harm the mycelium, so be careful.

Trim the shiitake mushrooms at the base of the stem using a clean knife or pair of scissors. Keep a little portion of the stem linked to the substrate to encourage additional fruiting.

Oyster mushrooms may be prepared using the same cutting technique as shiitake mushrooms. Cut them off at the base of the stem when they reach the proper size.

Morel Mushrooms: Be cautious not to disturb the neighboring soil while cutting morel mushrooms by cutting them at ground level.

Harvesting Suggestions

Harvest mushrooms when they are still tender and fresh for the best flavor and texture.

To prevent bruising or damage, use caution while handling mushrooms.

Since leaving mature mushrooms on the substrate might inhibit the appearance of new flushes, regular picking is required.

Remove any rubbish or damaged mushrooms to maintain the growing area sanitary and productive for the next harvests.

Chapter

5

More than the Basics

Congratulations! Your trip into the fascinating world of mushroom growing has already started. You've learned the fundamental techniques, gained an understanding of mushroom reproduction, and grew your first batches with success. However, the moment has come to advance and look at subjects unrelated to the basics. In this chapter, we'll examine complicated concepts and procedures to increase your comprehension of mushroom cultivation.

Understanding Substance Formulations

Up until now, you've presumably been working with simple substrates like vermiculite or brown rice flour. You'll practice advanced mushroom growing while learning how to make custom substrate compositions. Your harvests will significantly increase if you modify your substrates to meet the particular needs of distinct mushroom species. You'll discover additions like coir, straw, and others that enhance the nutritional value of your substrates.

Temperature and Humidity Regulation

Consistent environmental conditions are necessary for mushrooms to flourish. Beyond the basics, you'll learn more about regulating temperature and humidity. Discover how to create the perfect microclimates for different mushroom species and why maintaining them is essential during the whole growth cycle.

The Raising of Certain Species

More species should be considered if you're growing mushrooms at a higher level. You may have started with well-known varieties like shiitake or oyster mushrooms. Learn about the unique requirements of many culinary and medicinal mushrooms, including Lion's Mane and Reishi. Discover the subtleties of each species and how to adapt to their unique needs.

Disease Management and Prevention

As you go further in your agricultural operations, difficulties like contamination and illnesses will undoubtedly arise. You'll learn how to identify problems early, take preventive actions, and apply workable solutions to sustain healthy mushroom growth.

Expanding the Production Scale

Are you ready to turn your pastime into a small business? We'll go through the methods and elements to consider when you raise your mushroom yield. Making the most of your workspace, managing bigger workloads, and looking into new markets for your products are all necessary for this.

Complex Methods of Cultivation

Examine cutting-edge cultivation techniques like cloning and strain isolation. You may distribute top-notch mushroom strains using these methods for consistent quality and yield. Modern methods like automated growth systems and fruiting chamber design will also be discussed.

Past Mycology

In addition to teaching you about the practical aspects of mushroom farming, this chapter will also introduce you to the fascinating topic of mycology. Discover more about the ecology and science of fungi to understand their role in nature and the larger implications of their research.

Building Community

Finally, we'll talk about how to work with other mushroom enthusiasts. These strategies could include engaging in online forums or joining local groups. Building a community may be fulfilling and can provide you with wise counsel and inspiration as you continue to expand your understanding of mushroom cultivation.

Thank you for completing this stage of your mushroom-growing project. You may discover this intriguing hobby's potential by going "Beyond the Basics." Remember that there is always more to learn about the fascinating and dynamic world of mushrooms. Put on your mycologist's hat, then begin the exciting next step in your mission to produce mushrooms. Enjoy your garden!

The Expansion of Your Mushroom Farm

Congratulations, fellow mycologist! Now that you've built a solid foundation in the art of mushroom cultivation, you're eager to learn more. Growing your mushroom farm might be an exciting and profitable endeavor. In this chapter, we'll look at the steps and techniques needed to successfully enhance your mushroom-cultivating efforts.

Identify Your Objectives

Before venturing into the world of scaling up, be sure your intentions and objectives are clear. What do you want to achieve by increasing your mushroom production? Are you open to providing local markets, restaurants, or farmers' markets with fresh mushrooms? You could be considering starting a small company or experimenting with various types of mushrooms. Knowing your objectives can help you develop your strategy and guide your decision-making.

Expanding Your Workspace

If you increase your mushroom output, you will need additional space to accommodate your growing activities. Check to determine whether your current system may be extended or changed to match your increased production goals. Many successful mushroom growers start in basements, garages, or additional rooms but quickly move to larger spaces, such as dedicated outbuildings or greenhouses, to satisfy demand.

Equipment and Supplies

Additional space calls for the use of additional equipment and supplies. To maintain a sterile environment when preparing the substrate, spend money on high-quality sterilizing equipment like pressure cookers or autoclaves. You'll also need more containers, substrate components, and spawn. Consider bulk buy options to save costs and ensure a steady supply of essential items.

Automaticity and Effectiveness

It may be possible to automate the management of larger amounts of mushrooms. Automation may improve the efficiency of procedures including substrate preparation, inoculation, and environmental control. Automated misting and humidity control systems, for example, may help maintain the right conditions for the growth of mushrooms, hence reducing the need for ongoing manual involvement.

Climbing Fruiting Chambers

As you scale up, you may need to alter your fruiting chamber design. Larger fruiting chambers or several chambers could be necessary to handle an increase in mushroom production. Ensure that the ventilation, humidity, and temperature are all under control in these spaces. Monitoring equipment like temperature and humidity sensors may be quite useful in maintaining the ideal development conditions.

Employees and Labor

More help may be required to manage the growing strain while scaling up. If your company grows quickly, consider hiring personnel or enlisting the help of friends and relatives. Proper training is required to ensure that everyone involved understands the need to maintain sterile conditions and follow cultivation procedures.

Marketing and Sales

The quantity of mushrooms you may sell will rise as you can grow more of them. To reach your target market, develop an effective marketing strategy. Consider selling your goods at farmers' markets, via local grocers, or directly to restaurants. Making links with local chefs and restaurants may lead to long-term cooperation.

Keeping Records and Ensuring Quality

Keep meticulous records of your expanding agricultural business. This requires keeping track of the operation, the environment, and any challenges or successes you encounter. You will be able to identify trends, address problems, and continuously improve your mushroom cultivation techniques if you keep correct data.

Although it could be challenging, expanding your mushroom farm can be incredibly rewarding. By setting up clear goals, investing in the right tools, and being committed to quality, you may grow your excitement for mushrooms. Remember that success in mushroom farming often requires tenacity, dedication, and a drive to learn from both successes and mistakes. As you go off on this intriguing mushroom farming journey, be ready to broaden your horizons and enjoy the bountiful harvests that are in store for you.

Investigating Different Species of Mushroom

In the fascinating world of mushroom gardening, there are many different types of mushrooms, each with unique characteristics, tastes, and growth requirements. For a successful journey into the area of mycology to begin, it is essential for a beginner in the art of mushroom growing to comprehend the diversity of these fungi. This chapter will delve deeply into the intriguing world of several varieties of mushrooms, studying their unique traits and sharing expertise on how to properly cultivate them.

The common button mushroom is called Agaricus bisporus.

The button mushroom, which is often bought in supermarkets, is one of the simplest mushrooms to produce. It's a great spot for beginners to start because of its tolerance and quick growth. The mild, earthy flavor of button mushrooms makes them a versatile addition to many different recipes.

Species of oyster mushrooms (Pleurotus): Both their gorgeous appearance and delicate, seafood-like flavor make oyster mushrooms highly regarded. They come in a range of colors, including white, gray, and pink. Since oysters are adaptable and can be grown on a variety of substrates, they are a popular choice for beginners.

The savory, deep taste of shiitake mushrooms (Lentinula edodes) is well-known in the culinary world. They are often used in Asian cuisine and have medicinal properties. Although growing shiitake mushrooms may be a bit more difficult than growing certain other varieties, the results are well worth the effort.

The enoki mushroom species Flammulina velutipes are recognized by their tiny caps and long, thin stems. They often show up in soups and salads and taste somewhat fruity. Enoki can be cultivated indoors under the right conditions, despite being a little more temperature-sensitive than other kinds of mushrooms.

The honeycomb-like appearance of the morel mushroom (Morchella spp.) has made it famous. Modern chefs are quite interested in utilizing them because of their earthy, nutty flavor. It may be challenging to cultivate morels, as they often need certain environmental conditions that are found in their natural habitat.

The "Lion's Mane" mushroom, Hericium erinaceus, is distinguished by its shaggy, white appearance and lobster-like taste and texture. They are also known for potential neurological and cognitive benefits. Growing Lion's Mane mushrooms may be entertaining and manageable for beginners.

Traditional Chinese medicine holds ganoderma lucidum, sometimes referred to as the reishi fungus, in high respect for its potential health advantages. They are often used to make medicinal teas and have a harsh, woody flavor. Reishi mushroom growing may need a bit more dedication and careful technique.

Selling and Buying Mushrooms

Congratulations on your success in growing mushrooms! As you've discovered throughout your journey through "Mushroom Cultivation for Beginners," growing mushrooms could be enjoyable as a hobby. But what if you want to go even further? What would occur if you had more mushrooms than you could ever consume and were thinking about selling them? The details of turning your cherished fungus collection into a side business will be covered in this chapter.

How to Prepare Your Mushrooms for Sale

Before you start selling your homegrown mushrooms, be sure they adhere to the strictest standards for quality and safety. Follow these steps to get your mushrooms ready for sale:

Harvesting: When the mushrooms are at their biggest and freshest, choose the optimum time to collect them. To gently remove them from the substrate or growing medium, use clean, sharp equipment.

Cleaning: Gently brush off any dirt or debris from the mushroom caps using a soft brush or a wet cloth. Avoid using water since porous mushrooms may absorb it and get spoiled.

Your mushrooms should be arranged in order of size, look, and quality. Customers like trustworthy, attractive mushrooms.

Packaging: Use sanitary, food-grade containers or packaging materials to protect your mushrooms during delivery and storage. The name of the mushroom kind and the expiry date should be written on the labels, along with the logo of your business.

Legitimate Matters

Before you begin selling your homegrown mushrooms, it's critical to be aware of any applicable municipal laws and limitations. This includes things like permits, licenses, health and safety regulations, and tax obligations. Consult your local authorities and, if necessary, get legal guidance to ensure that you are operating within the law.

How to Find Your Market

Choosing your target market is a crucial first step in selling your mushrooms. Think about the following choices:

Local Farmers' Markets: Local producers may sell their products, including mushrooms, at several farmers' markets. This could be a good place to start.

Ask local restaurants and chefs whether they would be open to incorporating fresh, locally sourced mushrooms in their dishes.

Online sales: Open an online store or use already established ones like Etsy or Farmers' Market Online to reach a wider clientele.

Programs for community-supported agriculture (CSA): Join forces with CSA programs that routinely provide participants access to fresh veggies.

Price of Your Mushrooms

Setting the right price for your mushrooms may be challenging. Consider factors such as your production costs, market demand, and the pricing provided by competitors. Make sure your product is marketable, competitive, and not underpriced.

How to Promote Your Mushrooms

Your mushroom sales enterprise relies on marketing for its success. Consider the following marketing strategies:

Branding: Create a unique brand for your mushroom business that includes a logo and packaging that reflect your commitment to quality.

Use social media to promote your company, provide information, and engage with potential customers. Facebook, Twitter, and Instagram are a few of these platforms.

Participate in local food-related events, join mushroom growers' associations, and network to meet potential clients and business partners.

Customer feedback: Pay attention to what they have to say and adjust your offerings accordingly.

Conclusion

As we near the conclusion of our journey through the fascinating world of mushroom cultivation for beginners, it is critical to evaluate the knowledge we have acquired and the opportunities that lay ahead. This book debunks what was once a mysterious process by extensively examining the art and science of mushroom production. I want to leave you with a few memorable life lessons and inspiring quotes before you close the book's last chapter.

Knowledge is the Key. We now know that the foundation of successful mushroom cultivation is education. Understanding the life cycle of the fungus, the many species that may be cultivated, and the environmental factors that influence growth are necessary for becoming a professional mushroom producer. Maintaining your education is crucial since it will aid you in achieving your goals.

Consistency and Patience: Both of these characteristics are necessary for the process of growing mushrooms. Failures are a crucial component of learning since not every batch will be perfect. Accept losses as opportunities to sharpen your skills and alter your strategies. Remember that even the most experienced growers were once beginners.

Environmentalism: Mushrooms are beautiful animals that are essential to our ecosystem. As you care for them, it's important to respect and understand their natural surroundings. To safeguard the environment and your mushrooms over time, you should put most of your work into employing morally righteous and environmentally friendly agricultural practices.

Sharing Your Work's Fruits: One of the joys of mushroom cultivation is sharing your crop with friends, family, and even your neighboring neighborhood. Whether you are producing for personal pleasure or are considering commercial farming, the satisfaction of offering people fresh, homegrown mushrooms may be quite satisfying.

Never Give Up Looking: The mushroom industry is huge and dynamic. You could wish to look into new species, techniques, and technological developments as your self-assurance and competence increase. A lifetime of learning and growth might be experienced as a mushroom farmer.

Join the Group: The mushroom-growing industry has a lively and welcoming community of enthusiasts, experts, and professionals. Consider joining local or online clubs, forums, or seminars for mushrooms to connect with others who share your interests. This network might be a precious source of knowledge, support, and motivation.

Finally, remember that growing mushrooms is more than just a skill or a hobby; it's also a journey of self-discovery, a connection to nature, and an endeavor to sustainably create food. No matter if you wish to grow mushrooms for your enjoyment or as a means of money, the information you have received from this book will serve as the foundation for your future success.

As you embark on your mushroom-growing journey and are successful in your pursuit of this useful and lovely pastime, I wish you success and endless pleasure. I wish you success in your mushroom farms and happiness throughout every leg of your journey. I appreciate you joining me on my fungal adventure, and I look forward to many more ripe harvests and delectable mushroom feasts in the future. Enjoy your garden!